Thinking as a Nurse

Bruce Austin Scott

iUniverse, Inc.
New York   Bloomington

Thinking as a Nurse

Email: bscott@deltacollege.edu

iUniverse books may be ordered through booksellers or by contacting:

iUniverse
1663 Liberty Drive
Bloomington, IN 47403
www.iuniverse.com
1-800-Authors (1-800-288-4677)

ISBN: 978-1-4401-6333-3 (pbk)
ISBN: 978-1-4401-6337-1 (ebook)

Library of Congress Control Number: 2009933812

Printed in the United States of America

iUniverse rev. date: 11/9/09

Consultants

Samantha Chan

With a bachelors from the University of California, Berkeley and great success in tutoring nursing students, Sam, a student nurse herself, gave a perspective that helped fine-tune the manuscript both in content and clarity.

Paula Thomson

As a high-achieving student who will enter the San Joaquin Delta College nursing program in Fall 2009, Paula gave me a number of ideas about study group practices. Her review improved and elucidated the book.

Ray Vining

A Shreveport, Louisiana certified registered nurse anesthetist and old friend viewed the content from the vantage point of a professional nurse in a specialty where critical problem-solving is a daily event.

Carol Lehn, my mother-in-law, whose lay perspective made this book more readable and understandable to the novice eye.

Nancy Scott Chaffin, my sister, photographed the cover scene, *Highland Trail*.

Contents

1

The Foremost Characteristic of Nursing

Nurses are certainly remembered for their care and regard for patients and these attributes are vital in nursing practice, but the foremost guiding characteristic of nursing must be *knowledge*. A particular body of knowledge is what distinguishes any profession or vocation.

The necessity of nursing knowledge and understanding exists because of a nurse's daily need to identify and solve problems. A patient is under the care of nursing because he has a problem or set of problems. It is the nurse's responsibility to know both the current problems and the problems for which the patient is at risk. The information required for this problem-solving is perhaps immeasurable—this is why nursing is a field in which learning has to be life-long.

Entry-level nursing programs prepare generalists. This practice requires that a significant volume of information is learned by student nurses. The importance of students having a high respect for nursing knowledge cannot be overstated.

This book's aim is to persuade, convince, and teach student nurses some of what it means to think as a nurse, not *like* a nurse, but *as* a nurse. Thinking as a nurse is a capacity that is not innate, though one person will have a greater talent for it than another. It is an ability to know what to look for, how to look for it, and, once it is found, how to respond to the finding. Thinking as a nurse is an ability that comes from acquiring nursing knowledge and the experience that is gained when the knowledge is applied in clinical practice. One cannot properly perform nursing without nursing theory, which itself is of limited value if it is not practiced.

Students have said to me, "I like being in the hospital but not in the classroom." The statement can have several meanings, but the one that is most worrisome is the message that the student does not draw the vital connection between nursing theory (what is taught in the classroom) and what is practiced in the hospital. For whatever reason, the student sees theory and practice as separate entities that do not have a strong and purposeful link. It is the responsibility of the nursing curriculum, the instruction of that curriculum, *and* the student to make those necessary connections.

A couple of months ago, I was putting in a shift as a staff nurse on a respiratory step-down unit when I heard a recent graduate pondering aloud concerns about her patient. "At three o'clock, he was alert and talking to me—now I can't wake him up. His breathing has slowed down, but his oxygen level is normal. I've ordered a stat ABG (arterial blood gas) and have a call into the doctor."

She was clearly thinking as a nurse, and I got to hear what she was thinking. Because she had assessed the patient earlier, she saw a change in his neurological status, connected the data of a decreased level of consciousness to gas exchange and serum glucose levels, and investigated both. When the ABG results came in, they showed that the patient was hypercarbic—the arterial carbon dioxide level was very high, and this event had depressed the patient's central nervous system. The situation required the placement of an artificial airway in the patient who was then transferred to intensive care and placed on a ventilator.

It was the ability of the nurse to use knowledge to solve problems that led to the successful treatment of this patient. Had the nurse seen the patient as simply sleeping and not noted the change in his breathing, or investigated the situation, the outcome may not have been successful. Daily, throughout institutions where nurses practice, situations similar to the one just described occur. This should teach us that knowledge and the ability to use it correctly is the starting point for effective nursing practice.

2

A Point of View Regarding Nursing and Medicine

Much has been made of the differences in nursing and medicine, almost to the point that nursing, in some corridors, has been seen to be at odds with medicine. If nursing is looked at from a non-political perspective, it is a partner with medicine. The intent of nursing is to prevent and cure of disease, as well as provide comfort in the patient's latter days.

It is advantageous to patients if the nurse understands medicine and its practitioners. A nurse knowing medicine does not mean that the nurse will encroach upon the physician's domain; it more likely means that the nurse's practice will improve.

A patient comes to the emergency department with heart irregularities and one of the physician's concerns is the patient's serum electrolyte levels. Lab tests are ordered. The patient's serum potassium level is dangerously elevated and the physician has to decide how to lower it. One method is to give insulin. What if the nurse caring for the same patient in the emergency department only knew insulin as a treatment for diabetes? What if that narrow knowledge or understanding of insulin caused the nurse to delay giving the patient the insulin because the nurse's thinking was, "The patient's not a diabetic—I'm not going to give insulin." Had the nurse been more interested and informed about medicine, she would have known that insulin not only transports glucose into cells, it drives potassium into them as well. The patient's care would not have been delayed. The point is, that knowing medicine does not mean the nurse *wants to be a doctor*—it means the nurse's capacity to help patients has increased.

Simply stated, physicians treat disease and nurses treat the effects of disease. Physicians diagnose disease; nurses diagnose responses to the disease. A patient develops weakness in the legs along with other problems, and the neurologist diagnoses the patient with multiple sclerosis. The nurse diagnoses the same patient with the problems associated with diminished mobility. The physician's care will focus on lessening the manifestations of the disease, as well as providing therapies that will reduce the progression of the disease or minimize its complications. The nurse will help the patient cope with the problems brought on by the disease.

Both practitioners are helping the patient within their realms or domains of practice. Nurses function under their state's nursing practice act, legislation that details what a nurse should and may do. It is a document about which all nurses under its jurisdiction should be informed.

The nurse practice act does not prohibit a nurse from knowing what physicians know. It does not place limits on what nurses can investigate. What typically limits the nurse is the nurse herself. This may be the result of nurses never being advised or encouraged to be curious about what it is that makes physicians tick.

One of the things I have wondered about as a nursing educator is why nursing courses rarely have medical books on their book lists. Nursing text books are not updated annually while some medical text books are. *Conn's Current Therapy*, a one-volume treatment guide is revised annually. As books go, it is going to have more up-to-date information about the treatment of a particular disease than a nursing text book that is revised every three years.

When should nurses learn to work with physicians and how should this take place? Since much of what nurses do in practice is affected by the physician's care of the patient, learning to work with doctors, listening to them, and understanding their approaches should take place early in the student nurse's education. Physicians should be viewed as allies and nurses should have a direct interest in their work and writings.

When I was working on a master's degree in 1981, I was in the Graduate Reading Room and picked up a recent copy of *The New England Journal of Medicine*.

I read an account of four men admitted to New York hospitals who had a never-seen syndrome that severely depressed their immune systems. I had neither seen nor heard of such a disorder in my reading of nursing literature. Today that disorder is commonly known as acquired immune deficiency syndrome (AIDS). Much information that directly affects nursing practice is going to appear in the medical literature before it shows up in nursing books or periodicals. This is a persuasive reason the medical point of view should be integrated into nursing curricula.

3

Professionalism, a Way of Life

Professionalism does not start at the time clock or end at shift hand-off; it is a way of life for those who enter it. When one is a professional, it is a full-time pursuit that frames the life of the individual and directs her way of being. *Mr. Hyde* prevented *Dr. Jekyll* from being a professional. It's impossible to have an existence that is in one instance characterized by professionalism, and in another, it's not.

The Sacrifice of Professionalism

An inherent characteristic of a professional is sacrifice. With the rewards come losses. Early on, the student nurse should understand this. There are experiences, responsibilities, and obligations that are a part of nursing that may not be appealing, and may even be repellant.

I was in a situation in which I was caring for a man who was going through alcohol withdrawal. He was hospitalized because of a mass in his abdomen and underwent extensive surgery. With a history of heavy, daily ethanol use, removing alcohol from his intake meant that he would both physiologically and psychologically experience the profound discomfort of withdrawal and extreme surgical pain. Despite receiving drugs that were aimed at relieving his pain and minimizing the manifestations of withdrawal, the patient became lividly discontent. He screamed nearly incessantly and disturbed other patients. Further, he made harsh, unkind, hostile, and threatening comments to the staff. It was a challenge to the nursing staff's professionalism as there were temptations to lash back at the patient, and even refuse to care for him. Professionalism prevents a nurse from firing back at an abusive patient. Furthermore, it is illegal to abandon a patient's care.

Nurses do not select their patients and may find themselves in situations in which their way of thinking, their values, and their own conduct are at odds with the patient's. In situations where the patient's expectations are reasonable, if concessions need to be made, it is the nurse who will make them, not the patient. The nurse should anticipate making sacrifices in deference to patients.

The Seriousness of Professionalism

I was once on a panel interviewing prospective nursing students. A question we asked all applicants was "Why do you want to be a nurse?" Most of the answers were of the I-want-to-help-people strain. Some were honest enough to say they thought job opportunities in nursing were more promising than other fields. But the answer that was most disappointing was, "I think nursing will be fun."

Fun as opposed to mundane or fun as in entertaining, lighthearted, and socially rewarding? Even in her youth when a nurse sees her life as a period with a focus on making friends, dating, going to parties, and, in short, *having a good time*, she must view her role as a nurse very seriously. For the patients, it can be a troubling time, a time when they may be facing a significant loss or losses. In her empathy, the nurse sets aside her need for pleasure, and seriously addresses the needs of her patient.

I was a day-shift nurse caring for an elderly patient whose room was across from the nursing station.

"Good morning, how did you sleep last night?"

"I didn't."

"Oh. I'm sorry, were you in pain?"

"A little bit, but not too much."

"Wonder why you couldn't sleep—I'll ask the doctor for a sleeping pill order."

"What you need to do is tell the night nurses to quit having parties."

In realizing the seriousness of nursing, the individual nurse should look at her own behavior and imagine how it may be affecting patients. It is important for nurses to conduct themselves with an emphasis on securing patients' trust and well-being, as well as preventing insult or offense to them.

The Prosperity of Professionalism

A profession and its participants improve with age. As experience is gained and more information is gathered, there should be evident changes that demonstrate the profession's greater benefit to its clients. The professional becomes an expert in her field or a segment of it. A nurse may be an expert in cardiology nursing, or in managing the care of children with cystic fibrosis. As a person gains tenure in nursing, she and her colleagues should see that she is more confident in her role, more adept at problem-solving and skills, and more commonly consulted.

A significant contribution a professional makes to nursing is her influence on others, particularly novices. This could go in one of three directions. One could promote professionalism among others by setting good examples, attending to detail, consistently meeting patient needs, and having a practice that is based on current standards.

A nurse could have a neutral effect, one that neither inspires others nor hampers them as professionals. She's seen as consistent and reliable, but dispensable (easily replaced by another average nurse).

Of course, in all fields, there is the representative who injures the profession by, for example, not taking her responsibilities seriously, making light of the important role of nurses, setting poor examples, and even undermining the work of other nurses. This could result from any number of factors; its correction is the responsibility of the individual nurse and her supervisors.

I was teaching in a nursing program in Los Angeles, and on days in which I did not have clinical, I would arrive in the parking lot at 7 a.m. Many days, I would be getting out of my car at the same time as a nurse who was a staff member from the unit where I taught clinical students. We would greet one another and I would think, "Doesn't his shift begin at six forty-five?" He would arrive on his unit 20 minutes late, get report, and then go downstairs to the canteen for breakfast, before ever seeing his patients. One day, I asked him if he and I could talk after work and he agreed. He was an affable young man, a recent graduate of the program where I taught.

"I want to just lay something out for you. I see you coming in late every day and getting breakfast before you check on your patients. Can you tell me about that?"

"Woops, I'm sorry,"

"Do you realize the effect that has on others, the patients in particular?"

"What do you mean?"

"Your being late makes the night shift nurses

late—they have to wait for you so they can report off. Then your patients don't see you the first time until nearly 8 o'clock. Do you think their needs can be ignored for that long because you want to come in late and eat breakfast?"

"Well, no one's ever said anything to me."

"No one, no other nurse, not your supervisor?"

"No, not anybody."

"Can you do me a favor, for your own good, and the good of the patients and other nurses?"

"Sure, what is it?"

"I want you to ask your co-workers to give you an honest assessment of your work. Tell them to be sincere and genuine. I also want you to ask the same of your supervisor. The people here like you, but they are letting you get away with behaviors that directly affect the patients. One day your failure to make the patients your primary concern may lead to a disaster. Your career is in jeopardy if you keep this up."

He was neither ungrateful nor resistant. I was surprised because in my experience, the first stopping place for many when criticism comes their way is *defensiveness*. I never noticed a change in him after that talk, and I don't know if he took my advice. I was hopeful that I would have had a more notable impact.

A point that may be made of this is that it is the

individual nurse who monitors and governs her behavior. If she is accurate in the assessment of herself,
what a physician once told me is true: "A professional
doesn't need supervision."

4

Thinking Conceptually

A concept is a term or statement that embodies lesser principles or ideas. It can be viewed as an umbrella for a group of related notions. Thinking conceptually means that the individual is able to understand more distinct concerns because she is *first* able to grasp the larger idea—the concept. Main concepts are typically supported by sub-concepts. An example of this is the sub-concept of *coagulation* supporting the main concept of *hemostasis* (circulatory stability).

Consider the concept of *danger*. Danger is a one-word warning that is easily understood to mean that beyond the danger sign is some form of harm. If a person understands that danger is something that can put her in jeopardy, it is not essential that she be familiar with the details of the risky situation.

A person walks by a chain link fence and a bold red sign reads, DANGER. A high-powered transformer could be on the other side of the fence, or a pack of vicious dogs. Either way, understanding the concept of danger prevents the person from going within or beyond the fence.

The Concept of Safety

In nursing, a dominant concept is safety. It's an ideal that should occupy the nurse's practice at all times. A technician from radiology calls the nurse, "I'm coming to pick up your patient to transport him to radiology for a series of X-rays." The nurse, knowing that her patient becomes rapidly short of breath with even minimal activity says, "Can those tests be done at the bedside with a portable X-ray machine?" She's thinking *safety*.

Much of nursing practice is dictated by concerns for safety. Annually, The Joint Commission releases its *National Patient Safety Goals* and nurses are expected to regard them in their daily practices.

The concept is safety. The details underlying safety include how to be safe when administering medications, how to ensure that abnormal diagnostic findings are responded to quickly, and how to continually provide a risk-free environment for the patient. The starting point for a nurse is to understand safety as a broad concept, and then apply it to every patient situation. Conceptual learning and thinking allow the nurse to maneuver through the unexpected events that can be common in nursing practice.

Following is a discussion of two vital concepts used in nursing practice.

The Concept of Hypoxia

Hypoxia is *inadequate* tissue oxygenation. It is often preceded by hypoxemia, a subnormal concentration of oxygen in the arterial blood. Because most diseases have at least some component of impaired tissue oxygenation, it is important for nurses to understand the concept of hypoxia. Grasping this concept means that much is understood about hypoxic disorders in terms of their pathology, manifestations, and treatment.

Once the nurse understands hypoxia, when she encounters a patient with a hypoxic disorder such as acute coronary syndrome (ACS) or pneumonia, she has a head start on managing the care of the patient. For example, the nurse knows that a characteristic of hypoxia is pain due to ischemia of the tissue. Pain in hypoxic states can signal that the patient is in trouble and needs rapid attention. If the nurse does not understand the relationship of pain and hypoxic states, she may either mistreat the pain or underestimate its gravity.

Suppose a patient with ACS reports chest discomfort to the nurse and the nurse only views the discomfort as pain rather than the result of myocardial ischemia (hypoxia). She may give a prescribed oral analgesic such as acetaminophen (Tylenol) or ibuprofen (Motrin) instead of a coronary artery dilator such as nitroglycerine. This improper decision-making hails from the nurse's unfamiliarity with the connection of ACS to hypoxia and its associated pain.

The Concept of Perfusion

A very useful concept in nursing is *perfusion*. All cells need oxygen and nutrition—they are provided these needs by perfusion. Perfusion is the process of the body's various forms of pressure forcing substances into the cells. Underlying the concept of perfusion are the sub-concepts of osmosis, diffusion, mean arterial pressure, gravity, and patency. Learning sub-concepts enhances a person's understanding of the lead concept. For example, knowing diffusion helps a person understand how impaired diffusion across the alveolar-capillary membrane lowers perfusion and leads to suppressed cellular oxygenation and tissue hypoxia.

Identifying Concepts

Concepts form the foundation of understanding diseases and disorders, as well as the signs and symptoms the diseases and disorders produce. Moreover, an understanding of related concepts helps the practitioner understand therapies or treatments for specific diseases and disorders. Early in a student's nursing education, she should learn to identify the concepts that, in a sense, summarize the content that is being taught. When covering diabetes mellitus, the concept may be *metabolism* or *cellular nutrition*. When the topic is renal failure, the concept upon which the student nurse focuses could be *fluid balance*. More than one concept may be linked to specific nursing information, and each concept may be useful in understanding several disorders.

In terms of studying diseases, concepts can be viewed as the *essential problem* of the disease. With rheumatoid arthritis (RA), for instance, the essential concept is *inflammation*. The concept that guides a person to understand RA is inflammation or the inflammatory process. In disseminated intravascular coagulation (DIC), the concept can be *coagulopathy*. A student will best understand RA and DIC if the student understands inflammation and coagulopathy.

Conceptual thinking eases the burden of learning and facilitates understanding. It takes away the agony of memorizing reams of facts that will only serve the learner for a short time. It makes education more interesting and useful in practice.

Let's take the simple concept of the *straight line*, the shortest distance between two points. Suppose for the purpose of a test, a student simply memorized the definition of a straight line and never thought of it conceptually. For that student, it was just a fact that needed to be stored in memory until the definition was no longer needed. Had it been conceptualized as a piece of information that has usefulness, the student would have more likely retained it. It could have been used to shorten a trip from one place to another, or for planning the placement of furniture in the home of a person with mobility problems. A golfer may strike a ball over a patch of trees to the green using the straight line concept.

So, the commission of student nurses is to gain an appreciation of concepts, to look for them in the midst of a whirlwind of material in the nursing curriculum, to ask nursing educators to identify and elucidate them, and ultimately, to use them in their clinical practices.

5

Thinking Empathetically

If a nurse can, for a time, set aside her own needs, ideals, opinions, and philosophies and understand the plight of someone else, especially her patients, she is exhibiting *empathy*. It is not an optional aspect of nursing—it should be a part of all nurse-patient interactions as well as those that relate to the patient. The ability to be empathetic has much to do with one's own values and experiences, and particularly her respect and understanding of others. Furthermore, it largely has to do with one's willingness to set herself aside for the benefit of others.

Very late one evening, long after visiting hours had ended at the hospital where I was practicing, a woman came to me and said, "I just arrived from Pennsylvania. I've been traveling for 16 hours. My brother is a patient here and he's dying. May I stay with him through the night?" Of course, my inclination was to unhesitatingly tell her yes for a lot of reasons: her brother was dying, she had traveled many miles, and who wouldn't say yes in this situation? However, the hospital policy was that patients in semi-private rooms could not have overnight visitors. I knew what the right thing to do was, but I had to do it within the policy of the hospital.

What concept or ideal led me to the problem's solution? Empathy. With the permission of another patient, other staff and I moved the woman's brother to a private room so that she could stay with him all night. That was very long ago, but through all these years of practice, it has served to remind me of the value of empathy.

Questions that Lead to Empathy

A nurse can check her empathy by asking herself questions. Examples of theses questions are:

1. "If I were in this situation, would I want to be treated the way I am planning to treat this patient?"

2. "If someone was watching and evaluating me right now, is this how I would be conducting myself?"

3. "Is my level of attentiveness to the patient, the level I would expect were I the one receiving care?"

Stereotypes

Deriving impressions about a person strictly from his appearance, living situation, associations, culture and ethnicity is stereotyping. It can be a conscious or inadvertent act. The root of stereotyping is found in a person's influences and life experiences.

In her ambition to *think empathetically*, a nurse should first be aware that stereotyping is part of one's humanness; it unavoidably happens to all of us, and to suggest to oneself that she does not stereotype is naïve and shows lack of insight.

When my family and I drove into our new Central California hometown on a very hot day in August, we came to a stop light in the downtown area. Our three children were in the backseat of the car, looking around, asking questions, showing a lot of curiosity when a tall, thin man ambled through the crosswalk. He was disheveled, unshaven and wore a full-length leather coat. One of the children anguished, "Lock the doors." She was stereotyping. The man never looked at us, never spoke a word, and was completely minding his own business. In less than a minute, we considered him a threat, someone we needed to be aware of.

It is important for a nurse to be aware of the influence her own stereotyping has on patient care.

"How does what I have preconceived about a person affect the way I take care of that person?"

"Do the track marks on his arms make me more casual about getting pain medication for him than I would otherwise?"

"Does the patient's age and appearance impact my responses to him?"

The ideal is to eliminate stereotypes—what is more realistic is to *work around* them—to prevent them from diminishing the nurse's practice. One may look at stereotypes as handicaps nurses must recognize in themselves. Once recognized, nurses prevent them from impairing their day-to-day care of a variety of patients.

The VIP Room versus The Ward

Some health care settings have areas that are designated for very important persons (VIPs)—individuals who perhaps are celebrities or big donors. At the same time, they may have areas in which three or more beds are in a room (wards). The unfortunate implication is that the care given to the patient in the VIP suite will be different than that given in the ward. Despite pressure from wherever it may come, unless a nurse is specifically assigned to provide private duty care to a patient, the care she gives one patient should not differ from that which she gives to another in terms of the dedication, regard, compassion, and attention to details.

6

Listening to Your Patients

I was passing by a room on a medical-surgical unit when I overhead a patient tell a nurse, "Those are not my pills. They are not the pills I take at home." As a nurse, I had previously heard that from patients—typically it means that the appearance of the pills given in the hospital differs from those taken at home (multiple manufacturers can produce the same drug). Nevertheless, a short time after hearing the interaction, I witnessed the nurse phoning the physician: "Dr._____, I'm calling to tell you that I gave the wrong medications to one of your patients."

"Those are not my pills" was the patient's warning to the nurse. Unfortunately, she did not heed his warning and gave him the wrong medications. She did not listen to her patient.

Thinking as a nurse includes valuing the role the patient has in his own care. It involves seeing the patient and his family as a part of the health care team, as part of the solution to the problems that unfold during the time the patient is under the team's care. Everything a patient tells the nurse has to be valued and taken seriously.

The Meaning Behind the Words

"Her pain medicine seems to be working for her," says one patient of her fellow hospitalized suitemate. The nurse turns, smiles and responds, "I think you're right, she always seems comfortable." Was the nurse listening to the meaning behind the words? Did she investigate to see whether the implication she thought she heard was actually there?

The patient's comment could have been her way of saying, "My pain medicine is not relieving my pain." One aspect of thinking as a nurse is listening for underlying, subtle, or hidden meanings in what patients are saying. Patients expect nurses to be perceptive.

At bedside change-of-shift report, the patient said to me, the on-coming nurse, "I'm not going to tell you to do your job." At that point, I assumed that what she meant was that her experience was that she needed to tell nurses to do their jobs—that we were not meeting her expectations of care. A short time later, I returned to the patient and said, "During report, you mentioned to me that you are not going to tell me to do my job. Are you finding that that is what you have to do—tell nurses how to do their jobs?" "Yes. I'm a social worker; I know what caregivers are supposed to do and that my clients should not have to tell me what to do in my job. I feel like I have to remind the nurses of their responsibilities." "I'm sorry that has been your experience. Can you tell me specifically what we are doing or not doing?"

The conversation yielded information that helped me and future nurses provide better care to that patient. It is important to listen to what patients are saying, to investigate the meanings, and to make adjustments in care based on findings.

Giving the Patient a Reason to Talk

Patients cannot be expected to lead the way in nurse-patient interactions. Though that may occur, it is not typical. It is the nurse who establishes an environment in which patients will want to be forthright in expressing themselves. Foremost in bringing this about is building trust and rapport with patients, and showing authentic concern for them and their needs.

Open-ended statements or questions to patients are more likely to get insight from a patient than short, closed-ended comments. "Is your breathing alright?" may elicit only a yes or no response while, "Tell me about your breathing" can provide more useful information.

Avoid putting words in a patient's mouth with comments such as, "You're not hungry, are you?" "Tell me about your appetite," would be a better way of gathering information from the patient.

Actions Speak Louder

It is commonly known that one's actions send a more accurate message than his words. With this truth, comes the necessity for nurses to expect that a patient's words may not match his expressions or body language. We need to attend to more than the patient's verbalizations. A stoic patient is grimacing when he moves and tells you he's not in pain. The teary-eyed patient tells you he's "okay, nothing's wrong."

It is not that nurses are expected to accurately interpret non-verbal messages; it's that they are expected to pay attention to and investigate them. The nurse sees a change in a patient's demeanor; she should ask a question that gives her insight into the cause of the change.

Care should be taken not to draw inaccurate conclusions from the patient's non-verbal cues—this can lead to an uncomfortable situation for both the patient and nurse.

"You're not eating; you must not like the food we serve."

"No, as a matter of fact, my doctor was just in here and told me not to eat, because they want to do a test on me that requires my stomach be empty."

A more effective statement from the nurse would have been, "Tell me why you're not eating your food."

The Pitfall of Assumed Relationships

Along the lines of nurses making assumptions regarding observations, an area where nurses must be careful is that of *assumed relationships*. I doubt any experienced nurse has not found herself in a situation such as the following.

"Oh, hello, you must be Mr. Miller's mother." "No, I'm his wife." This can result in a faltering of the nurse-patient rapport because the nurse assumed a relationship and insulted the patient's wife. The ideal is to never draw such conclusions because invariably at some point the nurse will be wrong—this can hamper nursing care. The notion that it's an innocent mistake that should be dismissed by the patient or his associates denies the nurse's empathetic responsibility. In situations where the nurse needs to know the relationship of another person or persons to the patient, such as in instances where confidential or sensitive information is being divulged, it is preferred that the nurse directly ask a question such as, "What is your relationship to the patient?" or "Tell me how you are related to the patient."

7

Intuition

A mother awakens abruptly without provocation. No noise in the house, no smells, no environmental changes. She checks on her only child—his forehead is hot. He's feverish. His body temperature is over 39 degrees centigrade. She gives her little boy a dose of ibuprofen (Motrin), rubs him with a cool cloth, and resolves to sit at his bedside the remainder of the night.

She was awakened by *intuition*, an innate sense that guides conclusions or suspicions—the notion that *something's not right*. Intuition leads to investigation which then may lead to intervention.

A subtle change in skin color, reduction in the vitality of the patient, an unusual word or statement, a quietness or stillness, maybe an odor—all of these can give a nurse a sense that a change has occurred, a change that should be investigated. A nurse's suspicion based on perhaps an unidentifiable difference is intuition, sometimes called the sixth sense. It is learned from experience, not textbooks.

In thinking as a nurse, the individual should first understand that intuition is a tool that needs to be recognized as a valid part of a nurse's repertoire. Because it is a suspicion, it cannot directly lead to intervention. If a nurse's intuition is that her patient's blood pressure is too low, she cannot go from that point directly to an intravenous fluid bolus. She stops to assess, and to look for data that will either confirm her suspicion or dismiss it. Directly beyond intuition lies assessment, not intervention.

How does a nurse develop her intuition ability? I don't think this can be consciously accomplished—it just happens. A starting point is the recognition of intuition as a part of nursing practice. It is unpremeditated. A nurse enters a room for one purpose and her intuition becomes the focus instead. Rather than ignoring what she *feels*, she acknowledges her intuition as legitimate and looks for tangible support for her sense that something is different, not quite right.

I was caring for a woman in her late 50s when her daughter and son-in-law arrived for a visit. I greeted them, told them who I was, and left the room. I remember distinctly thinking there was something amiss with the son-in-law, something that I could neither put my finger on, nor ignore. I turned around and went back into the room thinking I was going to act like I forgot something. When I walked into the room, the son-in-law was sitting in a chair looking forlorn, dazed, and worried. I said, "Something's going on with you, isn't it?"

"I think you're right. I feel strange."

"What's wrong? Can you be specific?"

"My tongue is getting bigger and my lips are tingling."

"Are you having trouble breathing?"

"Sort of. I'm getting scared."

I turned to his wife who was beginning to panic. "Where were you before you came here?"

"We were at Red Lobster."

"Do you think your husband is having reaction to something he ate?"

By that time, the young man's face was flushed and his lips were swollen. He was breathing more rapidly. I called the charge nurse and told her to stay with the young man while I got a wheelchair. We rushed him to the ED where he was treated for a severe hypersensitivity. He was unaware of his allergy to shellfish and had eaten shrimp at the restaurant before visiting his mother-in-law.

I had never met nor heard of the patient's son-in-law, knew nothing about him, and yet intuition led me to pay attention and follow up on a visceral feeling. I could have been completely wrong—that is a risk the nurse takes when she follows her intuition. One nurse will be better intuitively than another, yet all nurses, especially as their time in nursing expands, will learn to give credence to their gut feelings.

8

Thinking Courageously

In the pilot episode of *Hawthorne*, a TNT Broadcasting series about nursing in a Richmond, Virginia medical center, a nurse caring for a young Iraq War veteran has an order to administer 16 units of insulin for a capillary blood glucose just over 200 mg / dl. The nurse recognizes the dose as unusually high and calls the patient's physician for an order confirmation. The physician lectures the nurse about challenging the order and instructs him to give the dose as prescribed. The nurse reluctantly gives the dose. Dramatically, the patient goes into cardiac arrest due to the "nurse giving an overdose." Television. Nevertheless, the depiction sent an important message to nurses—be courageous. If your knowledge and experience causes you to second-guess something, don't get bullied into going against your judgment.

The role of advocacy in nursing has many faces—sometimes a nurse advocates for something, and at other times she will be oppositional in her advocacy.

One Saturday morning several years ago, I assumed the care of a patient who worked for an airline. During a turbulent flight, a carry-on fell from an overhead bin and landed on her foot. She had been in severe pain for weeks before she underwent surgery to repair the damage. Postoperatively, she was receiving morphine sulfate and her agony continued. Her pain had prevented her from sleeping and she was in tears. "It's like I'm not getting any medicine—I don't think it is having any effect." It could have been the dose, the frequency, or the drug itself. It was not a problem I could solve independently. I called the surgeon who increased the dose of the morphine. The change in dose did not improve the situation, so I called the pharmacy for a pain consultation. A pharmacist specializing in pain management evaluated the patient and called the surgeon with his recommendation. The analgesic was changed to hydromorphone (Dilaudid) and within minutes after receiving the first dose, the patient's pain began to disappear. She was insensitive to morphine sulfate and advocacy helped reveal that.

Managing a stand-alone brain injury unit in the 1990s, I became entangled in a failed advocacy. We moved from one location to another, and in the new location, there was one private room. Because none of our eight patients needed to be isolated, any one could have been placed in the private room. It was my decision who would be placed there. I didn't have a plan, so I waited to see which family would request the room once they were informed of the 9-bed facility's layout. A husband of a patient approached me and asked that his wife be in the private room. I granted his request—"When we move, I'll make sure she's in that room." There was one open bed, and a few days before we moved to the new setting, a case worker for the facility called me and said a new patient was being admitted and would be in the private room.

"What? I've already promised that room to another patient."

"Well, you're going to have to un-promise it. It is part of the arrangement for moving the new private-paying patient to our facility."

"I can't do that—I already assured the family that she would get the private room."

"Quit beating a dead horse—it's done and you're going to have to let them know that you made a mistake."

"No, I didn't make a mistake. I'm going to refer the family to you so you can explain this whole thing to them."

"No, you're not; you are going to do your job and tell them that the private room is reserved for someone else. That's it."

I eventually went over the case worker's head, but my argument fell on deaf ears. I had to ignominiously give the news to the patient's husband who rightfully railed against me.

I should have consulted others before I made the decision about the private room. Things do not always go the way the nurse wants them to, and lessons can be learned from both successful and failed advocacy. The point is, thinking as a nurse includes having the courage to be the patient's advocate.

9

On Defensiveness

The need to explain, offer an excuse, find a cause or deny responsibility for an act is *defensiveness*. Though we all need to defend ourselves or our positions from time to time, a general posture of defensiveness will thwart a nurse's thinking. Defensiveness diminishes a nurse's ability to be objective about herself, to make changes in her practice, and to appreciate criticism and learn from it. It can lead to others' inordinate carefulness with the nurse out of fear they will hurt her feelings or injure her ego. In general, people don't like confrontation and if they feel that bringing something to the attention of a defensive nurse will lead to conflict or insult, they will avoid the topic. Because of her own defensiveness, a nurse who needs and could benefit from another person's observations will not be informed of the observer's thoughtful and useful criticism.

I was making patient assignments for my students early one morning when the activity of a staff nurse caught my attention. She was going from room to room without washing her hands, touching all sorts of contaminated objects, rubbing her nose, and adjusting her clothing and hair. I was in a quandary about saying something to her because I was an outsider of sorts, and could be perceived as inappropriately intruding into the affairs of others. Then without washing her hands, she was about to draw medicine into a syringe and give it to a patient. I couldn't refrain myself: "When was the last time you washed your hands?" "I can't remember," she responded. "You've been touching your face and other contaminated objects, and now you're going to prepare a medication?" "But I haven't touched a patient since I washed my hands." She became defensive, almost indignant with me, and the conversation went poorly.

Perhaps my approach was not ideal, but my intent was for the well-being of the patients. I would have been remiss to not have addressed my observation with the nurse. Her response to me can naturally make me less likely to speak to her again, if what I want to say to her may cause her to become defensive. I may have felt like the loser in the situation, but the person who lost was the one who defends herself when she is clearly wrong.

Criticism Does Not Have to be Constructive

If the constructiveness of criticism is what determines its merit, the criticism may never reach its intended recipient.

The American culture protects its citizens from emotional strife. We have Little League games in which the score cannot be kept, rules against using red ink to grade students' papers, and a common expression, "There's no such thing as a stupid question."

> A woman, in her ninth month of pregnancy is browsing in a maternity shop when a fellow patron approaches her, "Are you going to have a baby?" (Forgive me; that's a stupid question.)

Along with these is the commonplace notion that criticism is only valid and useful if it is *constructive*. In other words, if a person presents an observation or complaint to another, it must be fashioned in such a way that it is clearly perceived as constructive and not judgmental or offensive. Rather that telling someone not to smoke, we say, "Thank you for not smoking." The strain is upon the conveyor of the criticism, not upon the one being criticized.

One may say that this approach makes for a more civil society. Actually, it makes for a less reality-based society, filled with people who feel violated and victimized by simple statements of fact. Though nursing is in the midst of this cultural phenomenon, we cannot let its practices prevent us from being real with one another.

Criticism is necessary for growth in the profession, and the focus should not be on how carefully it is delivered, but that it is delivered at all. Nurses need to know the truth about themselves and their practices, and we must be strong about both delivering criticism and receiving it.

I was in a faculty meeting some years ago when the astonishing news was given that a recent graduate from the program had erroneously given a patient intravenous pancuronium (Pavulon), causing the patient's death. Faculty members loudly gasped, and afterwards several offered comments such as, "I knew she was going to end up doing something like that." I was new on the faculty and neither knew nor had derived an impression of the student. After hearing their surprising comments, I spoke up, "If you knew that she was going to endanger the community, why did you let her graduate?" There was silence. There is a great reluctance in nursing education to be honest with students out of fear that students will bring a grievance against the faculty member. Privately, faculty members will express reservations about individual students, but publicly will do nothing about them.

When I was on the nursing faculty at the University of Alabama, a student in the program arrived at clinical with black smudges on her forehead. According to her instructor, it looked as though she had accidentally either smeared make-up, or had touched something dirty, and transferred it to her face without knowing it. "There's something on your face. You should go to the lady's room and wash it off before clinical," the instructor advised. The student recoiled, "It's Ash Wednesday." "What do you mean?" the teacher questioned. The student made a big fuss about the event, accusing the instructor of religious discrimination, when the reality was that the instructor was ignorant of the Roman Catholic practice. The teacher had made an honest mistake, yet the student was intent on discomforting the teacher.

Fear of retribution and litigation undermines nursing instructors' willingness to provide their students valuable, edifying, and authentic evaluation. The onus does not rest upon the teacher alone—it is also the students'. Teachers must criticize, and students must expect and accept their criticism. This is an inseparable part of learning to think as a nurse.

10

Everything You Do Affects Your Patients

Patients are the central focus of nursing practice. This daily realization is a vital part of thinking as a nurse. It is not an overstatement that every step a nurse takes in her practice can either have a beneficial or injurious effect on her patients (and other nurses' patients as well).

One of my students was caring for a patient who was in his first postoperative day. He was having severe surgical pain and was receiving continuous hydromorphone (Dilaudid) by way of a patient controlled analgesia (PCA) device. The machine contained a large syringe of the drug and delivered a prescribed dose continuously, as well as patient-requested doses at 10-minute intervals. As the drug infused, the syringe emptied to an eventual point where it needed to be replaced by a fresh syringe that was stored in the medication-dispensing cabinet. When the syringe was nearly empty, the PCA machine alarmed the nurse who then had a short period of time to replace it. Often, because of other responsibilities, the nurse cannot immediately change the syringe when the alarm activates.

Regarding my student's patient, there was the typical delay in responding to the alarm. When the matter was addressed and the primary nurse went to retrieve the replacement syringe, there were no Dilaudid PCA refills in the dispensing cabinet. As a result, the pharmacy had to be called and instructed to deliver a replacement syringe. There was a 40-minute wait for the replacement syringe. The nurse who removed the final syringe from the dispensing cabinet was to have notified the pharmacy of the need to replenish the Dilaudid syringe supply. She did not fulfill that responsibility, and her behavior caused a patient to unnecessarily experience pain for over 40 minutes.

A converse situation that I recently learned of was a situation in which a young man's mother was rushed into an emergency department (ED) with a life-threatening event. The young man, acutely concerned about his mother's care and well-being, became angry when he thought that there was not a high enough urgency attached to his mother's case. The nurse that was caring for the mother was incapable of dealing with the son. A male nurse in the area, knowing the potential volatility of the situation and its impact on the care of the young man's mother and other patients in the ED, befriended the young man, pulled him aside, and talked to him about what was taking place. He explained how the young man's mother was being cared for and what the intent of the ED staff was. The genuine concern the nurse showed toward the young man allowed the nurse caring for the mother to be more effective, and likely abated problems for others in the ED. Further, the young man's experience on that day led him to pursue nursing as a career. He recently completed a nursing program and was esteemed by his instructors.

Turning the Focus Away from Yourself

With many years as a clinical instructor in nursing programs, especially with new student nurses, I have noticed their anxiety and uncertainty about their presence in the hospital. Certainly, their angst comes from inexperience and limited skills, but, in my opinion, it mostly comes from their focuses upon themselves. It's not selfishness—it's self-preservation. Student nurses have told me that they feel like "imposters," that they "don't belong here." It's a completely understandable point of view for them to have, and one should have empathy toward them, but the problem with it is that their emphasis is upon themselves in a place and time when it should be directed toward the patients. The student's level of self-awareness can actually be a hindrance to her progress and an impediment to the patient's well-being.

As an Army Nurse Corps Officer, I was assigned to practice in a 6-bed intensive care unit (ICU) at a medical center. Not all of the nurses with whom I worked wanted to be critical care nurses—it was just the way the Army worked—you go where you're assigned. From the first day of her role in the ICU, one of my colleagues verbalized and demonstrated uneasiness and anxiety in the unit. She undervalued her own capability, questioned most of her decisions, and continually lamented her situation to fellow nurses. We thought of her as a basket case. As time passed, she did not gain in confidence, but, because she had no other option, she hung in there.

Then one day, a patient she was caring for converted into a lethal cardiac rhythm—a circumstance that required an immediate response from the nurse. She saw what was going on, probably knew she needed to act, but instead started emptying the bedside trash. Her perception of herself in that emergency situation was her role was to take out the garbage. She had not developed in the setting to the point that her focus was more on her patients than herself.

It is a challenge for a student nurse to see herself as an important part of the clinical setting. It is, of course, partly due to her sense of incapability, lack of confidence, or perhaps her uncertainty that the path she has chosen is the right one. Nevertheless, with all of the elements affecting the student nurse's view of herself, early on, she has to understand that she is the least important person in the patient-nurse dyad. If on a given day, the nurse is unable to make her patients her priority, her focus, and her motivation, that is a day when the nurse cannot be optimally effective in her nursing care.

Manifestations of the Patient-First Way of Thinking as a Nurse

How does a nurse know she's participating in a way of thinking that puts her patients' needs before her own needs? Following is a list of some of those evidences.

1. She volunteers to help peers with their work.

2. She often asks her patients about their needs.

3. She's conscious of avoiding activities (gossip, unit chit-chat, surfing the web at work) that distract her from her patients' needs.

4. She looks for ways to bolster the practices of colleagues.

5. She invests more than just wage-earning time to make herself a better informed nurse.

11

Ingraining the Right Way

For a nurse's thinking to be beneficial to her patients, it must be the *right* thinking. It must come from a scientific foundation, one built upon findings that are contemporary and shown to be effective in both promoting wellness and preventing harm.

A nurse I was working with some time ago misread a poorly-written physician's order and administered 100 units of long-acting insulin when the prescription was for 10 units. For a number of reasons, it was a stunning mistake. The likelihood of giving 100 units of insulin in a single dose is so remote, so rare, and so unusual that the dose alone should have alarmed the nurse and provoked her to collaborate with others before giving the injection. The outcome of her error led to interventions for the patient that would have otherwise been unnecessary.

Current nursing practice mandates that all insulin doses be double-checked by another nurse. Before giving insulin, the dose must be confirmed by a second licensed nurse. This contemporary practice is the *right way*—it's not optional, and if done correctly reduces mistakes such as the one my co-worker made.

In many circumstances, there is no one right way of safely meeting the needs of patients, however, there are certain precepts that always hold true and will never change. Adherence to these precepts will help lead the nurse to proper thinking and performing.

Safety

To protect her back from injury during a dressing change on a bedridden patient, the nurse elevates the full bed. So she can manage the dressing change, she lowers an upper side rail. She prepares her dressing change field, removes the old dressing, and a voice from out in the hall yells, "There's a phone call for you." She tells the patient, "I have to get that—I'll be right back." She turns and leaves the room.

The nurse overlooked the precept of safety and increased the patient's risk for infection (leaving the wound uncovered) and risk for injury (leaving the side rail down with the total bed elevated). There are a number of ways she could have maintained safety. She could have postponed the phone call and finished the procedure, had another nurse take over the procedure altogether, or instructed someone else to answer the phone. Safety should always be paramount in a nurse's thinking.

Asepsis

Preventing patients from harm includes taking measures that will reduce their risk of infection. Thinking as a nurse involves a persistent awareness of ways that a nurse can optimize a patient's resistance and limit his exposure to pathogens. Of course, hand cleansing sits atop a list of things nurses must do if their practices are to respect asepsis. Less obvious nursing actions include making proper room assignments in the hospital, avoiding the use of community objects in isolation rooms, teaching the patient and his associates about infection control, and ensuring that patients get adequate daily calories.

Patient Preeminence

When a nurse enters the clinical setting, she realizes that it's not about her at this point—it's about the patients. Certainly, there needs to be a level of self-awareness in the nurse—her role, her performance, her effect on patients, however, it cannot override the care of the patients.

In September, 1974, because of foggy conditions, the crew of a flight landing in Charlotte, North Carolina was using an instrument approach rather than the visual approach that would be employed under clear conditions. The plane crashed, killing 74. In its investigation of the cockpit voice recorder, the

National Transportation Safety Board discovered that during the landing, the crew responsible for the landing of the aircraft was engaged in non-essential conversation including politics and automobiles. They had tragically allowed their focus to drift away from the plane's passengers to themselves.

A drastic example to make a vital point—the nurse must remember her reason for being where she is and act in a way that shows it. She establishes in her mind that patients are vulnerable and need her undistracted attention.

Privacy and Confidentiality

"Please pull the curtain," she scolded me. She should not have had to remind me of that. As a nurse, I am obligated to continually protect the privacy and confidentiality of my patients. Showing unwavering respect for this aspect of their care guides a nurse's daily thinking and problem-solving. It has the benefit of outwardly showing empathy toward patients—this can elevate the rapport between nurse and patient as well as the patient's trust and responsiveness to the nurse.

Objectivity

Nurses have a responsibility to be unhampered by prejudice and preconceptions. The ideal of entering a nurse-patient relationship with a *clean slate* can be challenging in certain circumstances; yet, it is not optional for the nurse. Nurses must view their patients as deserving the highest level of care the nurse can provide, regardless of the nurse's temptation to make judgments about the patient. It is ingenuous to believe that persons do not judge other persons (We make judgments about food, clothing and housing—how could we not make judgments about people?). However, it's improper, inappropriate, and unprofessional for a nurse to tailor her care based on these judgments.

12

The Smartness of Teamwork

Because nursing is a profession that largely depends on its members to function in teams, it is vital that student nurses have an inescapable view of the value and necessity of teamwork.

The Benefits of Teamwork

1.   Teamwork brings different sets of eyes to clinical situations. It maximizes problem-solving because more persons are seeing and evaluating the events.

2.   Teamwork promotes role modeling in nursing. It presents situations where one nurse can learn by observing another nurse in action.

3.   Teamwork preserves the individual's physical functioning. It reduces the incidence of injuries to the nurses.

4.   Teamwork promotes time management. Work-

ing together allows nurses to keep pace with daily routines and manage unexpected clinical events.

5. Teamwork shows patients there is a broader interest in their well-being. Nursing looks more like customer service when teams are directly involved in the care of patients.

6. Teamwork allows for fine-tuning of individual nursing practices. One nurse sees another nurse perform a certain way and can offer pointers which will improve the practice of that nurse.

Consequences of Not Using Teamwork

1. Missed observations. Without teamwork, details or events that would ordinarily be noted may be overlooked when working alone.

2. Injuries. Moving a patient by oneself has a greater likelihood of causing injury to the patient and/or nurse than when it is being done as a team.

3. Reduced enthusiasm. For most nurses, one of the joys of practice is working alongside other professionals. When nurses work alone, outside of teams, that sense of satisfaction is diminished or disappears. In the long run, it can have an ill-effect on patient care.

4. Changed attitudes. Nurses who are accustomed to working in teams may feel alone in that ethic. It can dampen their resolve and reduce the quality of the care they give.

Does Teamwork Need to be Formalized?

Do nurses need to work in a setting where team nursing is the mode of patient care delivery in order to function as teams? No. Teamwork can purely be due to the effort of the nurses assigned to a unit. Certainly, the leadership of a unit should set the tone both through policy and role-modeling, but the ones who are likely to make it work are the nurses at the bedside.

I have worked with any number of nurses whom I would characterize as *natural team players*. They consciously look for ways in which they can aid others. I remember a time when I was clearly running behind schedule. Without my asking or even letting it be known that I was not on time, one of my colleagues did the capillary blood glucose tests on two of my patients and came to me with the results. "I could see you were running behind, so I did your blood sugars—do you want me to give their insulins?" That seemingly small circumstance made an inspirational impact on me as a nurse—it heightened my belief in the importance of *voluntary* teamwork in nursing.

Thinking as a Team Member

In developing oneself as a team member, there are thoughts that can move the individual more and more in the direction of team work.

1. Being helpful to other staff will likely inspire them to help me when I need them.

2. If I help others with their care, the quality of the care for all patients on the unit should improve.

3. When I involve myself in areas beyond my own assignment, I will gain experience and learning that I would otherwise miss.

4. Because the patients will see a team effort aimed at promoting their well-being, their trust in the nurses will be enhanced.

5. The teamwork reputation elevates the statue of the nursing unit and improves recruitment of qualified staff.

6. There are few and rare reasons not to employ teamwork.

13

Patho(physio)logy

Pathophysiology is the study of the changes in normal bodily function that lead to disease. It is looking at disease from the perspective of altered physiology. Pathophysiology manifests the ideal that the best way to fix a problem is to attack its cause. If the cause of a subnormal serum potassium level is vomiting, yes, replace the lost potassium, but treat the vomiting by determining what the anatomical or physiological cause of the vomiting is.

Built into the curricula of medical education is the study of anatomy and physiology, while nursing curricula are devised with the assumption that student nurses have completed the sciences before entry into nursing programs. Medical education uses the terminology of *pathology* with the implication that its students have an understanding of physiology; nursing uses the term *pathophysiology* with the supposition that student nurses either do not have an adequate understanding of physiology or need a review. Either way, it is important for health care practitioners to know normal physiology and understand how altered physiology causes disease.

The primary reason it is necessary to understand both normal and abnormal physiology is that this will lead to more accurate treatment. A patient reports to her nurse that she is having trouble "getting air." "When I walked to the bathroom and back, I got winded and now I can't catch my breath." The nurse calls respiratory therapy with the expectation that the patient will receive a nebulized bronchodilator. The respiratory therapist auscultates the patient's lungs and tells the nurse, "Her lungs are clear except in the bases where the sounds are inaudible. The patient does not need respiratory therapy."

The nurse reports the patient's symptoms to the physician who orders a stat chest X-ray. The chest X-ray results show the patient has bilateral pleural effusion. The space between the parietal pleura and visceral pleura (pleural space) is occupied by serous fluid that is putting pressure on the lungs and reducing lung capacity. This is the reason for the patient's dyspnea. The physician orders a diuretic and schedules the patient for a thoracentesis. The treatment is based on the pathology that led to the shortness of breath.

Treating manifestations (signs and symptoms) certainly has its benefit. A person has a severe headache that is making her incapable of even simple activities such as making breakfast before work. Her physician prescribes an analgesic and at the same time refers her to a neurologist who will investigate the pathology or cause of the headaches. Repetitive treatment of manifestations without vetting their origin could lead to a worsening or irreversible progression of the disease or diseases that caused the manifestations.

Nurses should conduct themselves in the same fashion—regard the signs and symptoms, but look for their causes. A patient has a black colored defecation—is it from bleeding in the gastrointestinal tract or the ferrous sulfate the patient has been taking?

The nurse's patient has an enlarged abdomen that is clearly not due to obesity. When the nurse gently taps the belly, a wave appears to move across the abdomen. Why is this an important finding by the nurse? Because the nurse understands pathology, she knows that her observations suggest that the patient has ascites (fluid collection in the abdomen) because of liver disease and/or protein deficiency. With her understanding, she knows that the patient is at risk for hypotension because volume has shifted from the circulation into the interstitium. She knows that if there is liver disease, the patient is at risk for bleeding because the liver produces most of the body's clotting factors. Her knowledge of pathology leads her to observations that can promote the care of the patient in terms of proper treatment and prevention of further problems. For example, when clopidogrel (Plavix) is scheduled for administration to the patient, the nurse withholds the dose because she knows that as an antiplatelet agent, it can exacerbate the patient's already increased risk for hemorrhage.

I once assumed the care of a patient with liver disease who had a catheter placed in his urinary bladder for the purposes of closely monitoring urine output. At the end of the previous shift, the urine collection bag had been emptied, so I was surprised when I assessed the patient early in my shift and found a bag full of urine. I assumed the patient had diuresed--I emptied the bag, and went on with my assignment. When I returned to the patient during routine rounds, I found the bag full again. At that point, I knew something other than diuresis was going on, so I emptied the bag again and called the primary physician. "What color is the urine?" he asked. I said, "Yellow—looks like normal urine." "Get a stat urinalysis and call me with the results," he ordered.

When the urinalysis results came in, I called the primary physician. "The urinalysis is not normal—it's loaded with protein." "I was afraid of that—I'll be there right away to see the patient. Make him NPO (nothing by mouth), monitor his blood pressure, and don't let him get out of bed."

The physician examined the patient and consulted a urologist who performed a cystoscopy on the patient and found that the tip of the urinary catheter had penetrated through the bladder and was serving as a conduit for the ascites fluid to depart the abdominal cavity. Within a matter of hours, the patient lost 18 liters of abdominal fluid. The urologist closed the opening in the bladder with sutures and the patient was transferred to intensive care where he recovered.

What part of the scenario demonstrates the importance of knowing pathology? First of all, the volume of urine is highly uncharacteristic, even when a patient is receiving diuretics. Secondly, it is abnormal for urine to contain protein. Protein is a large molecule that cannot normally pass through the glomerulus into the collecting tubules of the nephron. Proteinuria is always an abnormal finding and in most cases would suggest a kidney disorder. The patient's history of liver disease and the physician's knowledge of liver pathology led him to correct conclusions.

Why did the physician order what he ordered? Because he knew the pathology of liver disease and its implications. If the liver is diseased and not functioning, it allows fluid to third-space into the abdomen. This shifts fluid from the intravascular space which reduces circulating volume, and subsequently, the arterial blood pressure. That's why he told me to monitor the patient's blood pressure. Because the physician knew that a drop in blood pressure reduces cerebral perfusion and increases the risk for syncope or vertigo, he instructed me to keep the patient on bedrest. Getting the patient up could have increased his risk for a fall and injury.

Knowing pathology leads to correct problem iden-
tification and treatment. It equips the practitioner
with the ability to see beyond signs and symptoms
that can sometimes mislead physicians and nurses.

In behavioral health, a rudiment of practice in
caring for persons with depression is that an upward
swing in the patient's mood may *not* be as promising
as it appears. Professionals discovered that as the person departs the sadness and disinterest in social interactions and becomes more alive, his risk for self-harm
actually increases. He now has the energy to do that
which he couldn't do during the nadir of his depression.

If the nurse does not understand the psycho-
pathology of depression, she may misunderstand the
patient's vitality, lessen her attention to him, and
perhaps allow him greater liberties than he can with-
stand. If her nursing care is not rooted in an understanding of the pathology of the illness, her decision-
making may be erroneous.

It should be an inescapable reality for the student
nurse that learning normal physiology is not just a
rite of passage or an obstacle for entry into a nursing
program—it is the vital precursor to understanding
abnormal physiology. Routine refreshing of one's fa-
miliarity with normal physiology will make discussion
of diseases more relevant. This is particularly true regarding the study of pharmacology.

Pathology and Pharmacology

Drugs affect physiological processes. For this reason, it is important for the nurse who is administering medications to know physiology. If a normal physiologic response of the sympathetic nervous system is to increase the heart rate, the nurse who gives a pro-sympathetic drug (adrenergic agonist) should know that she must observe the heart rate before and after giving the drug. If the nurse does not understand the sympathetic response and the adrenergic agonist's affect on the heart rate, she may erroneously give a drug such as dopamine to a patient who is tachycardic.

Bronchioles, the airways that deliver and remove gas from the alveoli, are affected by a number of pathological processes, including asthma, bronchitis, and hypersensitive (allergic) reactions. Very early in her nursing education, the student nurse understands the role of bronchioles in the sustaining of life. Narrowed or obstructed bronchioles lead to poor gas exchange and can put the patient in severe jeopardy. Understanding this pathology and drugs' affect on it, especially in tenuous situations such as an acute asthmatic episode, is necessary for optimum nursing judgments and actions.

Acetylcholine and beta2 receptors affect the diameter of bronchioles. Acetylcholine, a neurotransmitter, activates the parasympathetic response which causes narrowing of bronchioles (bronchoconstriction) while stimulation or agonization of beta2 receptors leads to dilation of bronchioles (bronchodilation).

A patient with a history of urinary retention is receiving routine doses of bethanechol (Urecholine), a cholinergic agonist (parasympathomimetic) which causes urethral sphincter relaxation and urinary bladder contraction. At the time a dose is scheduled, the patient tells his nurse, "I'm noticing that it's not so easy to breathe—I'm having trouble getting air in. Can you call my doctor?" The nurse responds, "I'll listen to your lungs, put you on some oxygen, give you your bladder medicine and then call the doctor."

Because bethanechol is a cholinergic agonist, it stimulates the parasympathetic nervous system. One of the consequences is bronchoconstriction. The nurse's reaction to the situation was suitable except for her decision to give the patient his "bladder medicine." It would have been in the patient's best interest for her to withhold the Urecholine because of its effect on the bronchioles. Knowing the physiology of airway response to cholinergic agonists would have improved the nurse's decision-making in this circumstance.

"I'm getting a migraine—can you give me my Inderal?" the patient exclaims to her nurse.

"Where is the pain and how do you rate it?"

"It's bad, across the front of my head—I'd say a 9 or 10."

"Okay, I need to check your blood pressure, pulse and listen to your lungs."

"Listen to my lungs? I said it was my head."

Propranolol (Inderal) is a non-selective beta1 and beta2 antagonist which can reduce the severity of migraine headaches. Because it is a beta1 antagonist, it reduces heart contractility and rate which lowers the blood pressure. Its beta2 effect can lead to bronchoconstriction because blocking beta2 receptors causes narrowing of bronchioles. The nurse knew these things which led her to her assessment choices. Had the patient had hypotension, bradycardia, or wheezes in the airways, the nurse would have withheld the Inderal and consulted the prescribing physician.

The greatest friend a nurse can have as she prospers in the role of administering medication is a strong understanding of the body's physiological processes.

14

Using the Nursing Process as a Guide to Clinical Activity

The most recognizable nursing tool for thinking as a nurse is the *nursing process.* It is a five-step mechanism going from the gathering of data to the evaluation of the success of the nursing care provided. The nursing process in an invaluable method of approaching nursing practice—one that becomes second-nature for many nurses.

A benefit of the nursing process is that it can guide a nurse's practice in more ways than patient-specific. I use the nursing process to organize my daily practice. When I begin a shift in the hospital, I start by gathering data (assessment). Before I am given report by the off-going nurse, I arrive on the unit early and make sure I know where the crash cart is, what the unit's call back number is (the number you give the physician's answering service if you need to talk to the doctor), and the codes for getting into the medication cart or medication-dispensing device (Omnicell or Pyxis). Patient data such as telemetry strips and daily diagnostic test results can also be gathered.

The pass-off report extends the data gathering as

I listen to and record the off-going nurse's account of the day. Then I do at least a cursory assessment of my patients paying particular attention to the problems that caused their hospital admissions. Admitted for a myocardial infarction—do they have chest pain or dyspnea? Hospitalized for a repair of a fractured hip— are they properly positioned in bed?

During my initial rounding of the patients, I am looking for problems. This represents the second step of the nursing process—diagnosis. In many ways, a nurse is a detective always looking for problems or potential problems. A patient is admitted for water intoxication and the nurse is looking for neurological signs and symptoms, knowing that water intoxication can cause cerebral edema (brain swelling). A patient says to a nurse, "I'm not going to be here tomorrow," and the nurse looks beyond the literal interpretation and says, "Tell me what you mean when you say, you're not going to be here." A nurse must appreciate that her existence as a nurse has much more to do with her progressing capacity to identify and solve problems than her technical or psychomotor skills.

Perhaps the most challenging step in the nursing process, in terms of putting it into action, is the planning step. If problems approached nurses one at a time, planning might be a mundane event. But rarely do problems get in line—they arrive in groups. The nurse's mission is to determine how and in which order the problems should be addressed. In the suc- ceeding chapter, there is a discussion on giving prob- lems proper priority.

The planning step is the one in which the nurse establishes patient-centered goals that then direct the decisions about specific interventions for the patient. A patient has a *cryptosporidium* infection that has led to frequent, watery diarrhea. The nurse's concerns for the patient relate to hydration, nutrition, and the in- tegrity of the skin. The goals will then develop from her list of concerns—prevent dehydration, malnutri- tion, and skin damage, or promote hydration and ad- equate nutrition while maintaining skin integrity. It is really the goals that dominate the nurse's thinking, because it is the goals which direct the nurse's deci- sions about the specifics of what should be done.

After planning, the nurse uses intervention. In the case of the water loss from the *cryptosporidium* infec- tion, which should the nurse do, stop the loss, replace the loss, or both? In terms of nutrition, how is that going to be maintained—orally or parenterally? And, what's the best way to protect the skin?

Once the nurse has intervened, she wants to know if what she has done worked. If it worked, to what de- gree did it work? This is evaluation. Evaluation looks at the patient-centered goals to determine whether they have been met. Evaluation directs decisions about care—should it continue as is or be modified?

Successful, effective nurses are so accustomed to using the nursing process that it becomes an unconscious undertaking. Day-in and day-out, the nursing process yields positive outcomes for the patients. This being the case, the student nurse should highly value the nursing process in her quest to think as a nurse.

15

Determining What's Most Important

Primarily because of the pace of nursing practice, a vital ability a nurse should have is being able to put things in order of priority. Nurses can be barraged with simultaneous situations requiring answers and decisions. How do they know in which direction to go first? There are a variety of mechanisms available to nurses which can lead them to the right decisions about what to do and when.

The Nursing Process

A secondary benefit of the nursing process is its use in directing the nurse's activities for groups of patients. The nurse learns to assess, diagnose, plan, implement, and evaluate her group of patients, and use her observations in arranging her activities through the shift. Supervisors, planning the events of a day, will use the nursing process to balance assignments among a group of nurses.

Assessment precedes intervention. A nurse sees what appears to be a lethal dysrhythmia scanning across the telemetry screen in the nursing station, grabs the crash cart, rushes to the patient's room, and applies the defibrillation paddles to the chest of the pa-

69

tient. "What the heck are you doing lady?" the patient yells. On the verge of shocking a stable patient, the nurse realizes she didn't assess him before attempting the risky intervention. Because a lethal dysrhythmia can lead to cardiopulmonary arrest, the first action the nurse should have taken was to *assess for responsiveness*. Even in the most urgent situations, some form of assessment comes before intervention(s).

Physiological Needs

A fellow nursing instructor said to me recently, "There's a short distance between compensation and decompensation." She explained that from the time a patient's body, especially his autonomic nervous system, responds to changes or threats (compensation), there is a limited amount of time before compensation is exhausted and the patient decompensates. Unabated, decompensation leads to further degeneration and death. This being the case, certainly a patient who exhibits signs and symptoms of compensation (increased heart rate and respiratory rate, for example), should be attended to quickly.

Recently I was assigned a group of four patients on a telemetry unit. After hand-off from the previous shift, I determined that the patient with the greatest need was a woman who was transferred from ICU that day. She was anemic and in a lot of pain. Within one hour of report, that changed.

A stable patient with a history of coronary artery disease who was waiting for an angioplasty told me she had chest pain. Her pressing physiological needs altered my priorities. After the administration of supplemental oxygen and a nitroglycerine tablet, her chest pain ceased. She continued to be my highest priority until shortly after dinner when a patient who had a myocardial infarction four days earlier vomited and became tachycardic—his heart rate went from 70 to 120.

Vomiting could be a result of lack of oxygen to the stomach because of reduced pumping capacity of the heart. The increased heart rate is a compensatory response to inadequate oxygen delivery to the body. The patient's vomiting and rapid heart rate caused me to shift my priorities again, because, as my peer put it, "There's a short distance between compensation and decompensation."

Except in circumstances where the patient's prognosis is terminal or there are extraordinary events which alter conventional approaches (disasters, physical threats to other persons), physiologic needs are the main means of setting priorities. The emergency department (ED) model of *threat to life, limb or major body function* is useful in settings beyond the ED. This emphasizes a nurse's need to appreciate and understand normal and altered body function, and be able to apply this knowledge to clinical situations.

Patient Stability

A stable patient is one who exhibits manifestations of recovery, or whose well-being is not declining. Unstable patients demonstrate changes that depict current or impending decline in their health. A postoperative patient whose arterial blood pressure is dropping, while his heart rate is accelerating, could be bleeding or in the early stages of shock. The stability of patients within a group determines the nurse's priorities. Naturally, the less stable patients, and those on the brink of instability are a higher priority in care decisions than stable patients.

Risk Levels

Patients are routinely assessed for a number of risks including risks for skin breakdown, falls, nutritional deficit, and thrombosis. The results of these evaluations can assist the nurse in making better decisions and setting more proper priorities. Risk assessment leads to prevention measures. These can then aid the nurse in establishing priorities while avoiding events that may hamper the flow of her work.

A patient with a small bowel obstruction is not able to eat and is undergoing gastric decompression by way of a nasogastric tube. She becomes confused and disoriented and dislodges the tube from her nose. Her nurse discovers the situation and notices that the patient is tugging on the IV through which the total parenteral nutrition (TPN) is infusing. The nurse sees the increased risks to the patient and realizes the circumstances have changed her priorities. At this point, her interventions will be aimed at preventing the complications for which the patient is at risk. This may include moving the patient to a room where she will be more easily observed by all staff.

Avoiding Prolongation of Care

An eager first-semester clinical student of mine arrived on the unit early one day when breakfast trays were being given out. He offered to help the nursing assistant and she gladly accepted. He went from room to room greeting the patients while he placed their meal trays on the over-the-bed tables. Shortly after, while I was at the nurses' station making my students' assignments, a physician entered the area and asked, "Who fed my patient?" At the time I thought the question had nothing to do with me because I was unaware that my student was passing out trays. Subsequently, I learned that a patient, who was scheduled for an endoscopy of the stomach and not supposed to eat, ate the food my student had given him. The kitchen staff erred in sending a tray for an NPO patient. The event caused the cancellation of the procedure and extended the patient's hospitalization at least one day.

In thinking as a nurse, one must consider the effect her care has on the length of time the patient will be hospitalized. Because of the inherent risk hospitalization has on patients (infection and loss of mobility as instances), a nurse's care should be directed at getting the patient out of the hospital, or care setting as soon as is feasible. A large part of this is patient teaching: instructing the patient to do such things as monitoring his own blood pressure, changing his own dressings, and safely getting out of bed. When setting priorities, the nurse must include length of hospitalization as part of her decision-making.

Pain

When one hears the words, "I've never suffered like this in my entire life," she will better understand the importance of pain being a criterion for setting priorities as a nurse. Aside from the anguish pain can cause a patient, it has multiple possible ramifications including delayed wound-healing time, depression, and impaired tissue perfusion.

Disease Transmission Prevention

Because the condition or diagnosis of one patient can affect other patients, this impacts a nurse's plan of care, particularly when it comes to the risk of disease transmission. When a nurse has to decide who to see first, the patient who is free of communicable diseases has priority over the patient with a communicable disease. It is derived from the precept *clean before dirty*. If other factors come into consideration, this means of decision-making may be overridden, but it must be addressed.

Assume that a nurse has a case-load that consists of a patient who is immunocompromised by a regimen of neoplastic drugs and a patient with *Clostridium difficile*, a communicable microbe that causes severe diarrhea. Ideally this assignment should be avoided, but for the sake of discussion, imagine it did exist. Given that both patients are stable, which should the nurse see first? The cleaner one, the one *without* a communicable infection. The reverse approach would jeopardize the immunocompromised patient.

16

The Distraction of Technical Skills

A nurse's hands can be more valued than her brain. This does not advance nursing as a profession, nor does it optimize the well-being of patients. Of course, the ability to accurately perform technical tasks, such as changing dressings or instilling eye drops in a fashion that will ensure patient safety, cannot be underappreciated. But when the activities of a nurse's hands become the primary focus, especially when they are the means of evaluating nursing practice, there is naturally a misconception, misunderstanding, and undervaluation of the nurse's capacity to think.

I was recently listening to a conversation on the radio between the moderator and a woman who had been laid off from her job at a bank. The woman said, "I'm willing to do anything for a job," and the moderator asked, "What are you willing to do?" The woman replied, "I can be a nurse." Why didn't she say, "I can be a pharmacist?" I'm afraid her answer came from her perspective that nursing is a skill-oriented profession in which its practitioners are persons who have learned how to perform a set of techniques. She must have been thinking, "I can learn techniques—I can be a nurse."

The public's perception of nursing is important because it affects their individual interactions with nurses. If we are only seen as technicians, patients may not share information with us—information that will lead to solving their problems.

It is not an intention here to examine how the public came to its perception; however, it is worth mentioning that one of the main reasons may very well be the way nurses portray themselves. At a nurses' pinning ceremony that I attended, there were two notable student nurse speakers. Both nearly exclusively discussed the technical aspect of nursing. It left me with the frustration, "This is the impact we made on our students?" A few weeks ago, I attended a skills day and moved from one station to another where the emphasis was technical activities, not cerebral exercises.

Perhaps this is a societal matter. How many celebrity athletes can you name? How many contemporary inventors can you name? It would not be surprising that you can name several athletes and no inventors. A person is more likely recognized for the way his body moves than the way his brain works. Translated into nursing practice, this means that a nurse will more often be recognized for her technical skills than her problem-solving abilities.

One day in the clinical setting, a student came to

me and said, "I'll need your help when I give the enema that's been prescribed." I said, "Okay, let's look at the doctor's order and discuss the situation." I wanted her to understand the reason for the enema before she performed it. We examined the patient's chart, and the order read, "Tap water enema, 30 milliliters every four hours." For three days, the nurses had been giving the patient one-ounce (30 milliliters) enemas every four hours. I asked the student, "Why is the patient getting these enemas?" She said, "I don't know." I told her to ask the primary nurse and get back to me. The student came back and said, "She's not sure."

From my nursing knowledge and experience, I knew this was an extraordinary situation both because of the small volume of each enema and the frequency of them. I could not think of one situation where this practice made sense. I told the student that we could not give the enema until we understood its purpose. The primary nurse became curious as well—it didn't make sense to her either, so she called the physician for an explanation. The physician discontinued the order and we never found out why the patient got those repeated small-volume enemas. It seems that for those three days, what dominated the situation were the technical skills of the nurses, not their abilities to think as nurses.

Professional nurses are necessary for their thinking abilities, their capacity to look at sets of data and draw accurate conclusions that will lead to solutions of problems. They are not necessary if all that is needed is a population of persons capable of performing a list of technical skills.

A commission to student nurses is to not let that happen. Certainly they must learn the proper performance of a variety of psychomotor skills, but much more important is the ability to accurately analyze situations based on the acquisition of a body of information. Let the brain outshine the hands in the pursuit of nursing practice.

17

The Impediment of Memorization

Memorization is fact accumulation. Through methods such as flash cards or listening to digitally recorded lectures repeatedly, the individual stores information in the memory. These facts are then used, usually at a specific time such as examination day. It is a common way of studying by many high-achieving students who are accustomed to making A's in nearly every course they take. Memorization rewards hard-working persons in most academic situations and settings. It can incline a student to think of herself as a highly intelligent and excellent student. Nevertheless, in a field in which the professional is called upon to routinely not just know information, but also use it, memorization can be a sunny day friend who never shows up when the clouds and thunder are approaching.

As a teacher of nursing, I do not embrace memorization, though I know it has its place, and its importance. It is helpful to memorize certain things—phone numbers, normal lab value ranges, drug names. Not everything can be reasoned out. In my experience teaching nursing for decades now, I see memorization as more of a foe than an ally. As a tool of learning, it does not prepare students to figure things out, to solve problems, or to make decisions based on groups of facts or findings. It gives the student an artificial sense of achievement, but does not fortify the person for the world of work where the phone rings with a situation that requires a decision, not the recitation of a list of memorized facts. Having a limited ability to memorize can be an attribute because it forces the individual to learn in other ways, ways that likely have greater usefulness in life than memorization does.

A comment I've heard from any number of students is, "I've never in my life done so badly on a test." It could be that the student is simply stating a fact, but more often, it's a condemnation of the test from a student who has been perhaps very successful in testing due to a talent for memorization. The test rewarded the student's memorization ability because it required knowledge of certain facts, but it let the memorizing student down when it posed situations in which the student needed to both *know* and *use* the facts.

Persons who learn primarily by memorization do well in situations in which the body of information needed to succeed is clearly outlined for them: lists, definitions, dates, equivalencies. They labor over the well-defined content until they have memorized it sufficiently to recall it for the test, provided the test does not surprise them and wander outside of that established block of data. Courses in which the instructor gives detailed study guides are the heyday of the memorizer. The teacher gave them all the facts they need: their commission now is to cram all of the facts into their brains before the test. Comprehensive final examinations are killers, because at that point, they need to go back and *re-memorize*.

Have you ever wondered why the straight A student in high school performed only average on the college entrance examination and the C student who barely slipped by grade-wise did exceedingly well? The C student couldn't or wouldn't memorize, but learned to think and solve problems. The ability to solve problems is largely what aptitude tests such as college entrance examinations evaluate.

I cannot number the times I have heard comments such as, "I'd rather have a C student at the bedside than an A student." I always recoiled at that comment thinking that an A student is more likely the well-informed one and the one who would have the wherewithal to handle clinical situations. But over time, I realized that most of what is on nursing tests is information that can be memorized, and making an A is likely to be an evaluation of one's ability to memorize, rather than one's ability to construct a correct response in a clinical situation.

It is not the student's fault that she has learned that memorization brings rewards and a sense of success. It's a system that for whatever reason didn't teach students to think. Thinking is something that has to be developed. The one thing that can most benefit a person in an academic setting is learning how to think, how to solve problems.

After boot camp in the Navy, I was sent off to Basic Electricity School where I sat at a cubicle eight hours a day until I learn the basics of electricity—what current is, which way it moves, how it is measured. Three of my buddies and I started the course at the same time. When each of us finished, we were sent to our next destination where we would learn electronics and how to fix broken equipment. I did well in Basic Electricity School—I learned the facts. And then I went off to fix broken equipment, to use the information I had learned, and I didn't do so well. My buddies all succeeded—they could fix what was broken, while I was more likely to worsen the situation. The lead instructor called me into his office and said, "You are way behind your classmates. If you don't catch up, we're going to send you out to sea to be a deck ape, a swabee." My ability to memorize had only gotten me so far. Fortunately, rather than being sent to sea to mop the decks of a ship, I was sent to San Diego where I learned to be a hospital corpsman.

An important step in getting away from the memorization quagmire is for the student to examine her motivation for being in nursing school. Is it to learn nursing so that she will be an effective practitioner, or is it to achieve the highest scores and grades in the courses? If it is the latter, the student may adhere to the memorization approach to her own disadvantage. Grades are not unimportant, but they are less important than learning. The ideal is for the student to set her sights on acquiring the theory of the profession in a fashion that will make her a necessary part of the clinical setting in which she works.

18

Buddy Study

Routine, serious get-togethers with a classmate or group can enhance the levels of success of nursing students. It's built on the axiom that "two heads are better than one." Typically, study sessions are formed from friendships, common clinical groups, or compatible schedules. The ideal is that groups will have rules and specific practices. Following are ideas about each.

Setting the Ground Rules

1. Though the group will inevitably have some social content, it should be understood that the purpose of meeting is to study nursing.

2. At some point, a leader should be identified. Often this happens naturally—someone displays leadership characteristics that fit the group.

3. Individual preparation should precede study sessions. No one should come ill-prepared expecting others to feed them what they should already know.

4. If there are disagreements about content (what was taught in class, for example), there should be an established way of resolving these differences. In any nursing class, the instructor should be asked, "In your class, what is the final authority, lecture or the book?"

5. During study sessions, make a list of questions for the instructor and address them in class, during the instructor's office hours, or via email.

6. The focus of each study session should be established. It is probably best to start each meeting with the material that is most challenging and least understood. Never study difficult content at the end of any session, whether it's individual or group.

7. It's good to start with an intent statement such as, "Today we are going to study..." and end with a summary statement such as, "This study session covered the topics of..."

8. It is most effective if a pattern of study develops; for example, start with defining important terms and concepts, and then discuss specific disorders or diseases.

Study Group Techniques

1. Develop a list of question stems such as, "What should the nurse do first," "What is the most common manifestation of..." "Which drug or drug class would most likely be given in this circumstance," or "Why is it important for the nurse to monitor...?"

2. Use lecture notes as the basis for questions. Turn statements into questions. For example, the statement, "The mean arterial pressure (MAP) is a measure of perfusion" can become, "What is a good indicator of perfusion?" or "What is MAP a measure of?"

3. Remember the way questions were asked on previous tests and use those styles for devising study group discussion and questions.

4. Set up clinical scenarios and talk about what the nurse should expect, monitor, treat, and prevent.

5. Use personal clinical experiences to give examples of how particular cases and situations were managed.

6.   What would the instructor think or do? Over
     time, members of the study group will gain un-
     derstanding of the teacher's point of view which
     will help them devise study group questions and
     inquiries.

19

Picking the Best Answer

Becoming a professional nurse includes the common-place occurrence of taking examinations. Because the National Council Licensure Examination (NCLEX) includes a high percentage of multiple-choice questions, it is essential that during nursing students' education, they learn how to answer these types of questions. Multiple-choice questions can be categorized into four groups: fact-based, comprehension, application, and analysis.

Seasoned students are experienced in answering fact-based and comprehension multiple-choice questions. Most prerequisite nursing courses expect students to learn facts and connect those facts together. Both of these expectations can be evaluated with multiple-choice questions. Though it is important for the student to *know* the facts and to be able to relate them one to another, fact-based, and comprehension questions do not evaluate the student's ability to use facts.

Types of Multiple Choice Questions

Fact-based Questions

Fact-based questions are important in nursing because they incite students to study details that are important in their practice.

What is the reason for once-daily dosing of aminoglycosides?
1. Toxicity is less likely
2. More compatible with home care regimen
3. Reduced risk of phlebitis
4. More frequent dosing is ineffective

Correct answer: 1

Though the task is to know the fact that once-daily dosing of an aminoglycoside reduces toxicities, a corollary benefit is that it can lead to further questions from the student. "How would the nurse know the dose was toxic in a particular patient?" "What are the evidences that the drug has become toxic?" "If it is discovered that a patient has an aminoglycocide toxicity, what should the nurse do?"

The handicap of fact-based questions is that they do not directly lead student nurses to solve problems.

Comprehension Questions

A question that requires the test-taker to connect pieces of data or information is a comprehension question.

In a patient receiving a moderate dose of dopamine (Intropin), which manifestation should the nurse expect to see?

1. Rise in urine specific gravity
2. Slowing of heart rate
3. Increased mean arterial pressure
4. Weakened peripheral pulses

Correct answer: 3

The question requires the student nurse to connect the drug dopamine and its *moderate* dose to its manifestations. The choices also require the student to know certain facts in order to rule-in or rule-out answers. Mean arterial pressure (MAP) is an indicator of perfusion and a moderate dose of dopamine should increase the MAP. If the drug affected renal function, which it should do since it increases perfusion, urine specific gravity would decrease. Since dopamine is a beta1 agonist, its effect on the heart rate would be to raise it. Increased perfusion makes pulses more easily felt, not less palpable.

In the question, the test-taker needs to connect a specific dose range of dopamine to the manifestations of its effect on MAP, renal function, chronotropy (heart rate), and pulse amplitude. Though the question does not require the student to solve a clinical problem, it evaluates her ability to draw conclusions from data. This is a skill necessary for problem-solving.

Application Questions

Well-constructed application questions identify the student's ability to distinguish from a set of quality choices. The question posits a clinical situation in which a decision needs to be made.

A nurse is instructed by a provider to inject 25 units of NPH insulin into a 50 mL bag of saline and give it intravenously to a patient over 1 hour. Which is most important for the nurse to do?
1. Check the patient's serum glucose level before giving
2. Challenge the provider's order
3. Ask the provider if it should be given by gravity or by pump
4. Advise the pharmacy to prepare the mixture

Correct answer: 2

A provider has written an order and the nurse needs to determine which step is most important. When making a decision about a provider's order, the first step is always to determine its safety. If safety is bypassed, all other decisions are illegitimate. The key to the question is whether it is safe to give NPH (intermediate acting insulin) intravenously. It is not. The only insulins that may be given intravenously are rapid-acting and short-acting. The correct answer is to challenge the provider's order.

I have used this particular question several times in a course I teach. Often students select "Check the patient's serum glucose level before giving" as their answer because they have learned how important it is to avoid giving insulin to a patient with hypoglycemia (serum glucose less than 70 mg / dl). When they pick this seemingly obvious answer, it is likely the result of not carefully reading and analyzing the stem of the question. Some students will challenge, "You tricked us." "That was a tricky question." Perhaps it was. Nursing practice can be tricky.

I was caring for a patient who was receiving intravenous narcotic analgesia by way of PCA. The liquid crystal display (LCD) on the PCA machine showed that she was getting the doses she was giving herself, yet her reports of pain suggested she was not getting enough pain medication. I called the physician and asked for an increase in the dose of the medication. He reluctantly gave me the order. I increased the dose as prescribed, yet there was no reduction in the patient's pain. Something was not right. I looked at the machine carefully and discovered that the medication syringe had the same amount of drug in it as it did when I assumed the patient's care. The drug was not infusing into the patient because of a machine malfunction, yet the machine's display said it was. *I was tricked.*

I called the physician to inform him of the finding and he reversed the previous medication order. I replaced the malfunctioning machine with a properly-functioning one and gave a prescribed bolus dose of the analgesic to the patient, set it on the proper dosing, and within a short time, the patient's pain was under control.

Well-constructed exam questions, perhaps perceived by some as tricky, can actually train students to be more attentive to detail. This can serve them well in clinical situations such as the one I experienced.

Analysis Questions

Test items that require student nurses to use multiple concepts in deriving accurate conclusions are analysis questions.

A patient with a newly applied cast on the left leg following a fibula fracture reports loss of sensation in the left foot. Pedal capillary refill is sluggish. In which position should the nurse place the leg?
1.   Slightly dependent
2.   Elevated at 15 degrees
3.   Elevated at 30 degrees
4.   Neutral

Correct answer: 4

The student nurse must understand that following an injury such as a fibula fracture, there is inflammation. The newly-applied cast may not be tight on the extremity when it is first placed, but swelling from the inflammation can cause the cast to become too tight. This causes pressure on the vessels and nerves. Subsequently, the complication of *compartment syndrome* can develop. The nurse's response is to reduce the risk of compartment syndrome and related damage. If the leg is elevated, gravity will lessen perfusion to the extremity—this is an incorrect response. Lowering the extremity will increase gravity and increase swelling—

also an incorrect response. The neutral position neither increases swelling nor reduces perfusion. Neutral is the correct response.

The concepts in play when making a decision about the question are bodily response to injury, pressure, inflammation, perfusion, gravity and positioning. The student nurse needs to be familiar enough with these concepts that she can use them to make proper clinical decisions. This is analysis.

The Best Answer

Multiple-choice questions that offer the greatest long-term benefit to nursing students are those that educate them to distinguish which is best in a group. Because the item may offer more than one *right* answer, the challenge is to select the *best* answer. This is perhaps one of the most difficult realities new nursing students face—a right answer is incorrect because it is not the best answer.

A nurse is caring for a patient who is in the immediate post-operative period following abdominal surgery. The patient has a history of coronary artery disease and develops a dysrhythmia. Which should the nurse do first?

1. Review the patient's lab results and medications
2. Administer prescribed nitroglycerine
3. Place the patient on supplemental oxygen
4. Call a rapid response and the physician

Correct answer: 3

In the above question, all of the answers have a degree of correctness for the situation. Because abnormal serum values such as potassium or calcium can cause heart rhythm irregularities, it is important for the nurse to check the patient's lab results. It may be necessary to give nitroglycerine to the patient if the cause of the dysrhythmia is myocardial ischemia. If the situation is one the nurse cannot resolve, it may be necessary to activate a rapid response. However, the correct response in the situation is to administer supplemental oxygen since it is known that one of the causes of cardiac dysrhythmias is hypoxemia. The *first* thing the nurse should do is give oxygen.

For some students, these kinds of questions lead to frustration and even a sense of injustice. They are accustomed to test items that have a clear-cut, distinct, singular right answer. The intensity of their study has at times made test-taking so easy and matter-of-fact for them that they know the correct answer before they finish reading the question.

Ideals that Promote Selecting the Best Answer

Certain aims or ideals can help student nurses develop in their skill at selecting the best answers to exam questions and in making the right choices in clinical situations. Following is a selection of those ideals.

1. Use your knowledge of basic life support as one means of understanding what is most important in situations where a patient's condition is declining. Airway, breathing, circulation (ABCs).

2. Realize that there is only one answer that will be accepted as correct even when all the answers seem right.

3. Understand patient needs from most important to least important as a means of improving your problem solving. The hierarchy of needs may be different from one situation to another, depending on the status of the patient. In a patient who is dying, the greatest need may be comfort, not circulation.

4. Study with the expectation that the purpose of your learning is to apply information, solve problems, and make decisions.

5. Identify concepts you have learned in understanding the situations presented on exams.

6. Employ the nursing process as a tool for decision-making knowing that assessment precedes intervention. Look before you leap.

20

Knowing Drugs According to Class

A surprising amount of a nurse's practice involves medications: determining whether they are safe to give, understanding their significance to the patient, knowing what time is best to give the medications, and monitoring the patient's response to them. With the variety of drugs a nurse can encounter in her practice, early in her education she should commit to a way of learning and remembering medications. The most compact way of doing this is to learn drug classes.

The drug classification method that is most useful is the one that describes the action of the drug: histamine blocker, opioid agonist, calcium channel blocker, as examples. Some drug classes have multiple drugs within them: the selective serotonin reuptake inhibitors (SSRIs) for instance. If a nurse sets out to learn drugs by attending to individual drugs, because of the innumerable drugs and annual addition of new drugs, the task may be too daunting. If she understands classes well and is aware which class a drug represents, she will already know much about the drug.

Physiology First

Drugs impact the body's physiologic functioning, therefore the road to understanding their actions begins at knowing how the body works. It is particularly important for the nurse to be familiar with the central nervous system (especially its autonomic branch), neurotransmitters, receptors, and hormones. Once normal physiology is understood, it is easier to comprehend the effect that drugs have on specific body functions. Examples of understanding normal physiology and its contribution to knowing drug classes follow.

The Hormone, Aldosterone

Aldosterone, a hormone secreted from the adrenal cortex, among other things, causes water retention by the body. If the body is poorly hydrated, one mechanism it has to remedy this is to reduce the amount of urine produced, thus retaining water. This is partly accomplished by aldosterone.

A number of drugs block the release of aldosterone. The classic example is spironolactone (Aldactone), a potassium-sparing diuretic. This drug is primarily given to patients to promote urine production when they are fluid-retentive. Drug classes such as the angiotensin converting enzyme inhibitors (ACEIs) and renin antagonists (RAs) also block aldosterone—

this contributes to the lowering of the blood pressure in persons with hypertension.

Opioid Receptors

Within the brain and spinal cord are opioid receptors that are responsible for conveying the pain message. If these receptors are bound, pain is diminished or eliminated. A class of drugs that bind opioid receptors are the opioid agonists. They are commonly used analgesics and include the drugs codeine, morphine sulfate, hydromorphone (Dilaudid), and fentanyl (Duragesic). It is most important for the nurse to understand the characteristics of the class, opioid agonists, before knowing the individual drugs. Knowing the class means understanding its effects, both those that are expected and those that are untoward. Most importantly, she should know that opioid agonists depress the central nervous system and can cause sedation and respiratory depression. This single fact has guided many nurses to make necessary abrupt decisions about their patients receiving opioid agonists.

Dopamine, a Neurotransmitter

There are a number of neurotransmitters in the body and a wide selection of drugs that impact them. One of them, dopamine, affects a range of bodily functions including cardiac activity, the way the body moves, and how a person thinks and behaves. Drugs that have an effect on dopamine are given for nausea and vomiting, heart failure, shock, schizophrenia, and Parkinson's Disease. The nurse's knowledge of dopaminergic drugs should begin with an understanding of the substance, dopamine. Other important neurotransmitters that are affected by medications are acetylcholine, serotonin, adrenaline, and norepinephrine.

The Problem with Broad Classifications

Oftentimes, before a student gives a medication to a patient, I will ask the student, "What class is that drug?" The student's answer will be a broad classification such as antibiotic, antihypertensive, or anticonvulsant. Though it is necessary to know broad drug classifications, it is a handicap for a nurse if that is the extent to which she knows drug classes.

I have given antihypertensive drugs to patients with low-normal blood pressures. Why? Because though the drug was broadly classed as an antihypertensive, it was being given as an afterload reducer. The purpose of giving that particular drug at that time was to reduce the patient's resistance to cardiac emptying by giving a drug that dilates arteries. This reduction in resistance eases the heart's workload, a tactic beneficial to patients who are recovering from a myocardial infarction or are experiencing heart failure.

I recall a nurse co-worker phoning a physician

because a patient she was caring for was to receive carbamazepine (Tegretol) and did not have a history of seizures. Tegretol is broadly classified as an anticonvulsant, however, it can be effective against the pain associated with diabetic peripheral neuropathy. The physician thanked the nurse for her concern and informed her of the reason the patient was to be given the drug.

Broad classifications do not, for the most part, give a strong enough sense to the nurse as to why the patient is receiving the specific drug. In particular, the classification of *antibiotic* does not. First of all, and this is extraordinarily important to be understood, antibiotics are for bacterial infections only and not all bacteria are sensitive to all antibiotics.

When our first child was an infant, she developed a middle ear infection. It was not until the pediatrician aspirated a substance from her middle ear and had it cultured that he knew what specific antibiotic would kill the causative microbe. That was after our child had completed three other antibiotic regimens.

Knowing that a drug is an antibiotic does very little to help the nurse understand what is going on with the patient receiving it. Even assuming that the patient has an infection can be incorrect as sometimes antibiotics are given prophylactically to prevent an infection rather than treat one.

The ideal is that nurses would be dissatisfied with

simply knowing drugs in terms of their broad classification. This approach will not advance their nursing
practice and benefit their patients.

21

Afterward

The immense responsibility a professional nurse has is highlighted by her daily need to solve patient problems. This book examined many of the tactics and essential skills necessary for consistent, accurate problem solving. The focus was on the cerebral aspects of nursing, partly because of the author's perception that the psychomotor emphasis in nursing is too prominent and may overshadow the cognitive component of nursing. Though accurate hands-on practice is undeniable in nursing, it must be understood, not as the essence of nursing, but as a tool that supports thinking as a nurse. When a nurse performs a technical skill, underlying her performance is the cerebral justification that tells her how and why the skill is necessary in solving the patient's problem.

Among the numerous facets of nursing practice, intellect, both practical and analytical, is most important. The ideal is that a nurse be well-rounded practitioner with all the necessary capabilities expected of a nurse. However, a reality of life is that sometimes a person can do a reasonably good job at something, even though that person doesn't have all of the characteristics expected of the role. Nursing is not exempt from this reality. Nevertheless in nursing, the one characteristic a person in the role cannot be without is the intellectual capacity to solve patient problems in the clinical setting. This is largely the dominant message of *Thinking as a Nurse.*